Created by <u>BabyDreamers.net</u>

Free Book Offer:

<u>Get How to be a Super Mom For Free</u>

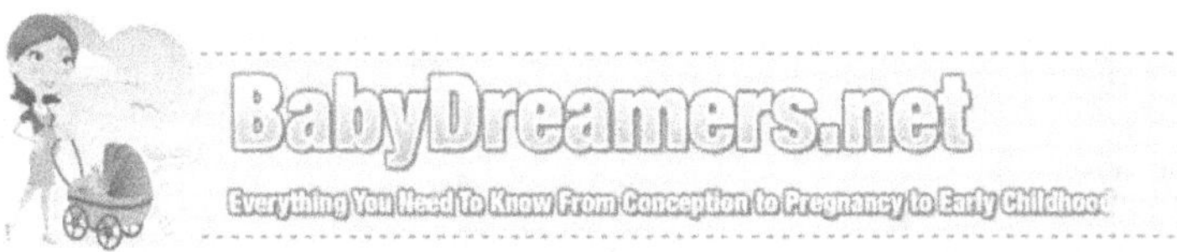

A Short Read is a type of book that is designed to be read in one quick sitting.

These no fluff books are perfect for people who want an overview about a subject in a short period of time.

Table of Contents

What You Need to Know About Tracking Your Ovulation

Tracking ovulation is a crucial step for women who are trying to conceive. Understanding the process of ovulation and knowing when it occurs can greatly increase the chances of getting pregnant. This article aims to provide essential information on tracking ovulation, including its importance for conception, various methods of tracking, and common misconceptions surrounding ovulation.

When it comes to conception, timing is everything. Ovulation is the release of an egg from the ovaries, and it typically occurs around the middle of a woman's menstrual cycle. By tracking ovulation, women can identify their most fertile days and plan intercourse accordingly, maximizing the chances of sperm meeting the egg. This knowledge is especially valuable for couples who are actively trying to conceive, as it can significantly increase their chances of getting pregnant.

There are several methods available for tracking ovulation. One popular method is basal body temperature charting, which involves measuring your body temperature every morning before getting out of bed. Another method is observing changes in cervical mucus consistency and color, as these can indicate the fertile window. Ovulation predictor kits are also widely used, as they detect the surge in luteinizing hormone that occurs prior to ovulation.

Additionally, smartphone apps have made ovulation tracking more convenient, allowing women to input data and receive predictions based on their menstrual cycle patterns.

Despite the importance of tracking ovulation, there are several misconceptions surrounding this topic. One common misconception is that all women ovulate on day 14 of their cycle. In reality, the timing of ovulation can vary from woman to woman and even from cycle to cycle. Irregular menstrual cycles can also pose challenges when it comes to tracking ovulation, but there are methods that can be adapted to accommodate variations in cycle length. Furthermore, not every woman ovulates regularly, as conditions like anovulation can affect fertility.

In conclusion, tracking ovulation is a vital aspect of family planning and conception. By understanding the menstrual cycle, utilizing various tracking methods, and debunking common misconceptions, women can take control of their reproductive health and increase their chances of getting pregnant. It is important to remember that every woman's journey is unique, and seeking medical assistance when needed can provide additional support and guidance.

The Menstrual Cycle and Ovulation

Understanding the menstrual cycle and the process of ovulation is crucial for tracking fertility and planning for pregnancy. The menstrual cycle is a complex series of hormonal changes that occur in a woman's body each month. It typically lasts around 28 days, although it can vary from woman to woman.

During the menstrual cycle, the body prepares for the possibility of pregnancy. The cycle begins on the first day of menstruation, when the lining of the uterus is shed. This is followed by the follicular phase, during which the ovaries produce follicles that contain eggs. One of these follicles will mature and release an egg in a process known as ovulation.

Ovulation is the key event in the menstrual cycle. It usually occurs around the middle of the cycle, approximately 14 days before the start of the next menstrual period. However, it is important to note that the timing of ovulation can vary from woman to woman and even from cycle to cycle. Tracking ovulation can help identify the most fertile days within a woman's menstrual cycle, increasing the chances of conception.

Why Track Ovulation?

Tracking ovulation is a crucial step for women who are trying to conceive or manage their reproductive health. By monitoring the menstrual cycle and identifying the fertile days, women can increase their chances of conception and take control of their reproductive journey.

One of the key benefits of tracking ovulation is the ability to identify the most fertile days within a woman's menstrual cycle. Ovulation typically occurs around the middle of the cycle, and tracking methods such as basal body temperature charting and cervical mucus observation can help pinpoint this fertile window. By knowing when ovulation is likely to occur, couples can time intercourse accordingly, maximizing the chances of conception.

In addition to increasing the chances of conception, tracking ovulation also allows women to manage their reproductive health effectively. By understanding the patterns and regularity of their menstrual cycles, women can detect any irregularities or potential issues early on. For example, irregular cycles or the absence of ovulation may indicate underlying hormonal imbalances or conditions such as polycystic ovary syndrome (PCOS). By tracking ovulation, women can identify these issues and seek medical assistance if needed.

Furthermore, tracking ovulation can provide valuable insights into a woman's overall reproductive health. Changes in cervical mucus consistency and color, as well as other physical and hormonal signs of ovulation, can indicate that the body is functioning optimally. Conversely, the absence of these signs may warrant further investigation into potential fertility concerns.

In conclusion, tracking ovulation offers numerous benefits, including identifying the most fertile days, increasing the chances of conception, and managing reproductive health. By utilizing various tracking methods and paying attention to the body's natural signs, women can take control of their fertility journey and make informed decisions about family planning.

Methods of Ovulation Tracking

When it comes to tracking ovulation, there are several methods available that can help women determine their most fertile days and increase their chances of conceiving. Let's explore some of these methods:

- **Basal Body Temperature Charting:** This method involves tracking your basal body temperature (BBT) every morning before getting out of bed. By noting the slight increase in temperature that occurs after ovulation, you can identify your fertile window. This method requires consistency and accuracy in recording your temperature.
- **Cervical Mucus Observation:** Monitoring changes in cervical mucus consistency and color can also provide valuable information about ovulation. As you approach ovulation, your cervical mucus becomes clear, slippery, and stretchy, resembling raw egg whites. This indicates that you are approaching your most fertile days.
- **Ovulation Predictor Kits:** These kits detect the surge in luteinizing hormone (LH) that occurs 24 to 36 hours before ovulation. By using urine or saliva samples, these kits can help pinpoint your fertile days. It's important to follow the instructions carefully for accurate results.

- **Smartphone Apps for Ovulation Tracking:** With the advancement of technology, many smartphone apps have been developed to assist women in tracking their ovulation. These apps use various methods, such as tracking menstrual cycles, BBT, and symptoms, to predict fertile days. They can provide reminders and personalized insights to help you plan for pregnancy.

Each method has its own advantages and may work differently for different women. Some women may prefer using a combination of methods to increase accuracy and reliability. It's important to find the method that works best for you and fits into your lifestyle. Remember, tracking ovulation is not an exact science, but it can provide valuable information to help you plan for pregnancy.

Basal Body Temperature Charting

Basal Body Temperature (BBT) charting is a popular method for tracking ovulation and understanding the changes in body temperature throughout the menstrual cycle. This method involves taking your temperature every morning before getting out of bed and recording it on a chart or in a smartphone app.

The purpose of BBT charting is to detect the subtle rise in body temperature that occurs after ovulation. Before ovulation, a woman's basal body temperature is relatively stable. However, after ovulation, the hormone progesterone is released, which causes a slight increase in body temperature.

To effectively use BBT charting, you will need a basal body thermometer, which is more sensitive than a regular thermometer. It is important to take your temperature at the same time every morning, before any physical activity or movement. This consistency ensures accurate tracking of your body's temperature changes.

When charting your BBT, it is recommended to use a graph or a charting app to plot your daily temperatures. This allows you to visualize the pattern and identify the shift in temperature that indicates ovulation. Typically, you will notice a slight drop in temperature just before ovulation, followed by a rise that persists throughout the second half of your cycle.

It is important to note that BBT charting alone cannot predict the exact day of ovulation. It can only confirm that ovulation has occurred after the fact. Therefore, it is beneficial to combine BBT charting with other methods of ovulation tracking, such as monitoring cervical mucus or using ovulation predictor kits, to increase accuracy and reliability.

By learning how to use basal body temperature charting, you can gain valuable insights into your menstrual cycle and increase your chances of conceiving. Tracking your BBT can help you identify the most fertile days within your cycle and optimize the timing of intercourse for pregnancy. Remember to be consistent, patient, and diligent in recording your temperatures to obtain the most accurate results.

Cervical Mucus Observation

Understanding how changes in cervical mucus consistency and color can indicate ovulation and fertility is an essential aspect of tracking ovulation. The cervix produces mucus that undergoes noticeable changes throughout the menstrual cycle, reflecting the hormonal changes that occur during ovulation.

By observing and tracking these changes, women can gain valuable insights into their fertility and identify their most fertile days. The consistency and color of cervical mucus can provide valuable information about the timing of ovulation.

During the beginning of the menstrual cycle, the cervical mucus is typically dry or sticky, making it difficult for sperm to travel through the cervix. As ovulation approaches, the mucus becomes more abundant, slippery, and stretchy, resembling the consistency of raw egg whites. This fertile cervical mucus helps facilitate sperm transport and increases the chances of conception.

Tracking changes in cervical mucus accurately involves regular observation and recording of its consistency and color. This can be done by checking the mucus on a daily basis and noting any changes in texture, stretchiness, and appearance. Some women find it helpful to use a chart or a smartphone app to record their observations and track their fertile days.

It's important to note that every woman's cervical mucus pattern may vary, so it's crucial to become familiar with your own unique pattern. By understanding the changes in cervical mucus and tracking them accurately, you can optimize your chances of conceiving and better plan for pregnancy.

Ovulation Predictor Kits

Ovulation Predictor Kits

Ovulation predictor kits (OPKs) are a valuable tool for tracking ovulation and increasing the chances of conception. These kits work by detecting the surge in luteinizing hormone (LH) levels, which occurs approximately 24 to 48 hours before ovulation. By identifying this surge, women can pinpoint their most fertile days and time intercourse accordingly.

OPKs are highly accurate in detecting ovulation, with a success rate of around 99%. They are easy to use and typically come in the form of urine test strips or digital devices. To use an OPK, simply follow the instructions provided with the kit. This usually involves collecting a urine sample and either dipping the test strip into the sample or using the digital device to analyze the hormone levels.

It's important to note that OPKs are most effective when used in conjunction with other methods of ovulation tracking, such as basal body temperature charting or cervical mucus observation. This comprehensive approach provides a more accurate picture of ovulation and increases the chances of conception.

When using OPKs, it's essential to track the results consistently and record them in a fertility calendar or app. This allows for better tracking of the menstrual cycle and identification of patterns over time. By understanding the timing of ovulation, couples can plan intercourse during the most fertile days, optimizing their chances of achieving pregnancy.

In conclusion, ovulation predictor kits are a reliable and convenient method for tracking ovulation and increasing the chances of conception. By understanding how they work and using them effectively, couples can take control of their fertility journey and make informed decisions about family planning.

Smartphone Apps for Ovulation Tracking

Smartphone apps have revolutionized the way women track their ovulation. These apps offer convenience, accuracy, and a range of features that make ovulation tracking easier than ever before. With just a few taps on your phone, you can keep track of your menstrual cycle, identify your fertile days, and increase your chances of conception.

One of the key features of smartphone apps for ovulation tracking is their ability to predict and notify you about your fertile window. These apps use advanced algorithms to analyze your menstrual cycle data and accurately predict when you are most likely to ovulate. This information can be invaluable for couples trying to conceive, as it allows them to plan intercourse during the most fertile days.

Accuracy is another important aspect of smartphone apps for ovulation tracking. These apps use scientific methods and data analysis to provide accurate predictions of ovulation. They take into account factors such as cycle length, basal body temperature, and cervical mucus consistency to determine your fertile days. By relying on these apps, you can have confidence in the accuracy of your ovulation tracking.

When it comes to popular options, there are numerous smartphone apps available for ovulation tracking. Some of the most popular ones include Clue, Flo, Glow, and Kindara. These apps offer user-friendly interfaces, customizable features, and the ability to sync with other health tracking apps. They also provide additional features such as menstrual cycle reminders, symptom tracking, and personalized insights into your reproductive health.

In conclusion, smartphone apps have made ovulation tracking more convenient and accurate than ever before. With their range of features, accuracy in predicting fertility, and popular options available, these apps are a valuable tool for couples trying to conceive. Whether you are just starting your journey to parenthood or have been trying for a while, consider using a smartphone app for ovulation tracking to increase your chances of conception.

Common Misconceptions About Ovulation

When it comes to ovulation, there are several common misconceptions that need to be debunked. Let's start with the belief that every woman ovulates. Contrary to popular belief, not every woman ovulates. Conditions such as anovulation can prevent ovulation from occurring regularly or at all. This is an important factor to consider for women who are trying to conceive, as it may affect their fertility journey.

Another misconception is that women always ovulate on day 14 of their menstrual cycle. While day 14 is often used as a general guideline, the timing of ovulation can vary from woman to woman and even from cycle to cycle. Factors such as cycle length and hormonal fluctuations can influence the timing of ovulation. Therefore, it's crucial to track ovulation using reliable methods to accurately determine the fertile window.

Irregular menstrual cycles can also lead to misconceptions about ovulation. Women with irregular cycles may find it challenging to predict when they will ovulate. However, tracking methods can be adapted to accommodate variations in cycle length. It's important to remember that irregular cycles do not necessarily mean a lack of ovulation. By closely monitoring changes in cervical mucus and using other tracking methods, women with irregular cycles can still identify their fertile days.

By debunking these misconceptions, women can have a better understanding of ovulation and make informed decisions about their reproductive health. It's essential to rely on accurate information and tracking methods to optimize the chances of conception. Now that we have cleared up these common myths, let's explore the signs and symptoms of ovulation to further enhance our knowledge of this crucial aspect of fertility.

Ovulating on Day 14

Ovulating on day 14 of the menstrual cycle is a commonly held belief, but it is actually a misconception. While day 14 is often used as a general estimate for ovulation, the timing can vary significantly from woman to woman and even from cycle to cycle. It is important to understand that every woman's menstrual cycle is unique, and ovulation can occur at different times for different individuals.

The menstrual cycle typically lasts around 28 days, with ovulation occurring approximately in the middle of the cycle. However, this is not always the case. Some women may have shorter or longer cycles, which can affect the timing of ovulation. Factors such as stress, hormonal imbalances, and underlying medical conditions can also influence the timing of ovulation.

To accurately track ovulation, it is essential to pay attention to the body's natural signs and symptoms. Methods such as basal body temperature charting and cervical mucus observation can provide valuable insights into the timing of ovulation. By understanding these signs and tracking them consistently over several cycles, women can gain a better understanding of their individual ovulation patterns.

It is worth noting that ovulating on day 14 is just an average estimate and may not apply to everyone. By debunking this misconception and recognizing the variations in ovulation timing, women can make more informed decisions when trying to conceive or manage their reproductive health.

Irregular Menstrual Cycles

Irregular menstrual cycles can have a significant impact on ovulation tracking. Women with irregular cycles may find it challenging to predict when they will ovulate, as the length of their cycles can vary from month to month. This unpredictability can make it difficult to accurately determine the fertile window and time intercourse accordingly.

However, there are methods that can be adapted to accommodate variations in cycle length. One such method is the use of basal body temperature charting. By tracking basal body temperature daily, women can identify the slight increase in temperature that occurs after ovulation. This rise in temperature can help confirm that ovulation has occurred, even if the cycle length is irregular.

Another method is the observation of cervical mucus. While the consistency and color of cervical mucus can vary throughout the menstrual cycle, women with irregular cycles can still track these changes to identify the fertile window. By monitoring changes in cervical mucus, such as the appearance of clear, stretchy mucus, women can determine when ovulation is likely to occur.

In addition to these methods, women with irregular cycles can also consider using ovulation predictor kits. These kits detect the surge in luteinizing hormone (LH) that precedes ovulation. By using these kits, women can get a more accurate prediction of when they will ovulate, regardless of their cycle length.

It is important for women with irregular menstrual cycles to be patient and persistent in their ovulation tracking efforts. By using a combination of methods and adapting them to accommodate variations in cycle length, women can still effectively track their ovulation and increase their chances of conceiving.

Not Every Woman Ovulates

Contrary to popular belief, not every woman ovulates. Ovulation is the release of an egg from the ovary, which is necessary for conception. However, there are certain conditions that can prevent ovulation from occurring, leading to difficulties in achieving pregnancy.

One such condition is anovulation, which refers to the absence of ovulation. Anovulation can be caused by hormonal imbalances, such as polycystic ovary syndrome (PCOS), where the ovaries produce too much androgen hormone, disrupting the normal ovulation process. Other factors that can contribute to anovulation include thyroid disorders and certain medications.

For women who do not ovulate regularly or at all, achieving pregnancy can be challenging. Ovulation tracking methods, such as basal body temperature charting and observing changes in cervical mucus, may not be effective in predicting fertile days. In such cases, seeking medical assistance from a fertility specialist is recommended. Fertility treatments, such as ovulation induction with medication or assisted reproductive technologies like in vitro fertilization (IVF), can help women with anovulation conceive.

Signs and Symptoms of Ovulation

When it comes to tracking ovulation, it's important to be aware of the signs and symptoms that indicate this crucial phase of the menstrual cycle. By understanding these physical and hormonal changes, women can better predict their fertile window and increase their chances of conception.

One of the key indicators of ovulation is changes in cervical mucus. Throughout the menstrual cycle, the consistency and color of cervical mucus can vary. However, during ovulation, the mucus typically becomes clear, slippery, and stretchy, resembling the texture of raw egg whites. This change in cervical mucus is a reliable sign that ovulation is approaching or already occurring.

Another common symptom of ovulation is ovulation pain, also known as mittelschmerz. This is a mild to moderate pelvic pain that some women experience during ovulation. The pain is usually felt on one side of the lower abdomen and can last anywhere from a few minutes to a few hours.

Ovulation pain can be helpful in tracking ovulation, as it often occurs around the same time as the release of the egg.

In addition to cervical mucus changes and ovulation pain, other signs of ovulation include breast tenderness and increased libido. Many women notice that their breasts become more sensitive and tender during ovulation. This is due to hormonal changes in the body. Additionally, some women experience an increase in sexual desire and arousal during this time, which can be attributed to the surge in hormones associated with ovulation.

It's important to remember that these signs and symptoms may vary from woman to woman and even from cycle to cycle. While some women may experience noticeable changes, others may not have any obvious symptoms. This is why tracking ovulation using various methods, such as basal body temperature charting and ovulation predictor kits, can provide a more accurate picture of when ovulation is occurring.

By paying attention to these physical and hormonal signs of ovulation, women can gain a better understanding of their menstrual cycle and fertility. This knowledge can be invaluable when trying to conceive or simply monitoring reproductive health. Remember, every woman's body is unique, so it's important to listen to your own body and track ovulation using the methods that work best for you.

Cervical Mucus Changes

Learn how to interpret the different types of cervical mucus and their significance in determining the fertile window and timing of ovulation.

Tracking changes in cervical mucus is a valuable method for determining fertility and predicting ovulation. The consistency and appearance of cervical mucus can provide important insights into a woman's menstrual cycle and help identify the most fertile days for conception.

Throughout the menstrual cycle, the cervix produces varying types of mucus, which can be categorized into different stages. At the beginning of the cycle, after menstruation, the cervical mucus is often minimal and dry. As the cycle progresses and ovulation approaches, the mucus becomes more abundant, slippery, and stretchy, resembling the consistency of raw egg whites. This fertile cervical mucus is the most conducive to sperm survival and can aid in the journey of sperm through the cervix and into the fallopian tubes.

By tracking changes in cervical mucus, women can determine their fertile window, which is the period when conception is most likely to occur. The presence of abundant, clear, and stretchy cervical mucus indicates that ovulation is imminent or has already occurred. This is the optimal time for sexual intercourse to maximize the chances of fertilization and pregnancy.

It is important to note that every woman's cervical mucus pattern may vary, and it is essential to become familiar with one's own unique pattern through consistent observation. Keeping a record of daily observations can help identify patterns and predict future ovulation cycles. Some women may find it helpful to use a fertility tracking app or a chart to document and interpret their cervical mucus changes.

In conclusion, understanding the different types of cervical mucus and their significance in determining fertility can be a powerful tool for couples trying to conceive. By tracking cervical mucus changes, women can accurately identify their fertile window and increase their chances of successful conception. Remember, consistency and regularity in tracking are key to obtaining accurate results. So, start observing your cervical mucus today and take control of your reproductive health!

Ovulation Pain

Ovulation pain, also known as mittelschmerz, is a phenomenon experienced by some women during their menstrual cycle. It refers to the mild to moderate abdominal pain or discomfort that occurs around the time of ovulation. Understanding ovulation pain can be helpful in tracking ovulation and increasing the chances of conception.

The causes of ovulation pain are not fully understood, but it is believed to be associated with the release of an egg from the ovary. As the egg is released, it may cause irritation or stretching of the ovarian wall, resulting in pain. The pain is typically felt on one side of the lower abdomen and can last anywhere from a few minutes to a few hours.

Symptoms of ovulation pain can vary from woman to woman. Some may experience a dull ache or cramping sensation, while others may experience sharp or stabbing pain. The pain may be accompanied by other symptoms such as bloating, nausea, or even light vaginal bleeding.

Ovulation pain can be a useful tool for tracking ovulation. By paying attention to the timing and intensity of the pain, women can gain insight into their fertility window. Ovulation pain usually occurs about two weeks before the start of the next menstrual period, which can help in determining the most fertile days for conception.

It's important to note that not all women experience ovulation pain, and its presence or absence does not necessarily indicate a problem with fertility. Additionally, ovulation pain should not be relied upon as the sole method of tracking ovulation. It is recommended to use other methods such as basal body temperature charting or ovulation predictor kits for more accurate tracking.

In conclusion, understanding ovulation pain, its causes, symptoms, and its potential role in tracking ovulation can be beneficial for women who are trying to conceive. By combining multiple tracking methods and paying attention to their body's signals, women can increase their chances of successful conception and take control of their reproductive health.

Other Ovulation Symptoms

When it comes to ovulation, there are more than just the obvious signs like changes in cervical mucus or ovulation pain. Many women experience a range of other symptoms that can indicate that ovulation is occurring. These symptoms are unique to each individual and can vary in intensity from woman to woman.

One common symptom of ovulation is breast tenderness. Some women may notice that their breasts feel more sensitive or tender during the fertile window. This is due to hormonal changes in the body and can be a helpful clue that ovulation is approaching.

Another sign of ovulation is an increased libido. Many women report feeling a surge in sexual desire during their most fertile days. This heightened libido is thought to be nature's way of encouraging procreation.

Some women may also experience a heightened sense of smell during ovulation. This can make certain scents or odors more noticeable and intense than usual. It's believed that this heightened sense of smell is linked to the increased levels of estrogen in the body during ovulation.

Lastly, changes in basal body temperature can also be a symptom of ovulation. Basal body temperature refers to the body's temperature at rest, and it can fluctuate throughout the menstrual cycle. During ovulation, a woman's basal body temperature typically rises slightly, indicating that ovulation has occurred.

It's important to note that these symptoms are not foolproof indicators of ovulation. Every woman's body is unique, and some women may not experience any noticeable symptoms at all. However, if you're trying to conceive or track your fertility, paying attention to these additional signs can provide valuable insights into your menstrual cycle and increase your chances of successful conception.

Factors Affecting Ovulation

Factors Affecting Ovulation

Ovulation, the release of an egg from the ovary, can be influenced by various factors. Understanding these factors is crucial for tracking ovulation and optimizing fertility. Here are some key factors that can affect ovulation:

- Stress: High levels of stress can disrupt the hormonal balance necessary for ovulation. Managing stress through relaxation techniques, exercise, and self-care can help optimize ovulation.
- Hormonal Imbalances: Conditions such as polycystic ovary syndrome (PCOS) and thyroid disorders can disrupt the hormonal signals necessary for ovulation. Addressing these imbalances with medical intervention can improve ovulation.
- Age: As women age, the frequency and quality of ovulation can decline. Women in their late

30s and 40s may experience reduced fertility due to age-related changes in their reproductive system.

- Underlying Medical Conditions: Certain medical conditions, such as endometriosis and pelvic inflammatory disease, can affect the health of the reproductive organs and interfere with ovulation. Treating these conditions can improve ovulation and fertility.

By understanding the factors that can influence ovulation, individuals can take proactive steps to optimize their fertility. Consulting with a healthcare professional can provide further guidance and support in managing these factors and increasing the chances of successful conception.

Stress and Ovulation

Stress and Ovulation

Stress is a common factor that can have a significant impact on ovulation, disrupt the menstrual cycle, and ultimately affect fertility. When the body is under stress, it produces higher levels of cortisol, a hormone that can interfere with the normal hormonal balance required for ovulation. This can lead to irregular or even missed ovulation, making it more difficult to conceive.

Managing stress is crucial for optimizing ovulation and increasing the chances of conception. There are several strategies that can help reduce stress levels and promote a healthier reproductive system. One effective method is practicing stress-reducing techniques such as meditation, deep breathing exercises, and yoga. These activities can help calm the mind and body, reducing cortisol levels and promoting hormonal balance.

In addition to relaxation techniques, maintaining a healthy lifestyle can also play a significant role in managing stress and optimizing ovulation. Regular exercise, a balanced diet, and sufficient sleep can all contribute to reducing stress levels and improving overall reproductive health. It is important to prioritize self-care and make time for activities that bring joy and relaxation.

If stress continues to be a major factor in disrupting ovulation and fertility, it may be beneficial to seek professional help. A healthcare provider or fertility specialist can offer guidance and support, and may recommend additional strategies or treatments to address stress-related fertility issues.

In conclusion, stress can have a profound impact on ovulation and fertility. By understanding the connection between stress and reproductive health, women can take proactive steps to manage stress and optimize ovulation. By incorporating stress-reducing techniques and adopting a healthy lifestyle, women can increase their chances of conceiving and ultimately achieve their family planning goals.

Hormonal Imbalances

Hormonal imbalances can have a significant impact on ovulation and fertility. Conditions such as polycystic ovary syndrome (PCOS) and thyroid disorders can disrupt the delicate hormonal balance necessary for regular ovulation.

Polycystic ovary syndrome (PCOS) is a hormonal disorder characterized by the presence of cysts on the ovaries. It can lead to irregular or absent ovulation, making it difficult for women with PCOS to conceive. PCOS is often accompanied by elevated levels of androgens, such as testosterone, which can further disrupt the ovulation process.

Thyroid disorders, such as hypothyroidism or hyperthyroidism, can also affect ovulation. The thyroid gland plays a crucial role in regulating hormone production and metabolism. When the thyroid is underactive (hypothyroidism) or overactive (hyperthyroidism), it can disrupt the hormonal balance necessary for ovulation to occur regularly.

It is important for women with hormonal imbalances to seek medical attention and work with healthcare professionals to manage their condition and optimize their fertility. Treatment options may include medication, lifestyle changes, and hormone therapy to restore hormonal balance and promote regular ovulation.

Age and Ovulation

As women age, their fertility declines, and this decline is closely linked to changes in ovulation. Ovulation, the release of an egg from the ovary, is a key factor in conception. In a woman's late 30s and 40s, the frequency and quality of ovulation can be affected, making it more challenging to achieve pregnancy.

As women approach their late 30s and 40s, the number of eggs in their ovaries decreases, and the remaining eggs may be of lower quality. This decrease in egg quantity and quality can lead to a decline in the frequency of ovulation. Additionally, hormonal changes that occur with age can disrupt the regularity of the menstrual cycle, further impacting ovulation.

It is important for women who are trying to conceive in their late 30s and 40s to be aware of these changes in ovulation. Tracking ovulation using methods such as basal body temperature charting or ovulation predictor kits can help identify the fertile days within the menstrual cycle and optimize the chances of conception. However, it is also important to keep in mind that age-related changes in ovulation may require additional medical assistance or interventions to achieve pregnancy.

Medical Conditions and Ovulation

Medical conditions can have a significant impact on ovulation and fertility. Two common conditions that can affect ovulation are endometriosis and pelvic inflammatory disease (PID).

Endometriosis is a condition in which the tissue that normally lines the uterus grows outside of it. This abnormal tissue growth can cause inflammation and scarring, which can interfere with the release of an egg during ovulation. Endometriosis can also affect the quality of the eggs and the function of the fallopian tubes, making it more difficult for fertilization to occur.

Pelvic inflammatory disease is an infection of the female reproductive organs, usually caused by sexually transmitted bacteria. PID can lead to inflammation and scarring of the fallopian tubes, which can block the passage of eggs and sperm. This can prevent fertilization from taking place and increase the risk of infertility.

It is important for women with these medical conditions to work closely with their healthcare providers to manage their symptoms and optimize their fertility. Treatment options may include medication, surgery, or assisted reproductive technologies, depending on the severity of the condition and the individual's goals for family planning.

Tracking Ovulation for Conception

Tracking ovulation is a crucial step for couples who are trying to conceive. By understanding and monitoring the timing of ovulation, couples can optimize their chances of conception and increase the likelihood of a successful pregnancy. Here are some key strategies for tracking ovulation to enhance the chances of conception:

- **Timing Intercourse:** One of the most important aspects of ovulation tracking is timing intercourse correctly. Couples should aim to have intercourse during the woman's fertile window, which includes the days leading up to ovulation and the day of ovulation itself. By having intercourse during this time, the sperm will have a higher chance of meeting the egg.
- **Understanding Fertility Windows:** Ovulation tracking can help identify a woman's fertility windows within her menstrual cycle. These windows are the days when she is most likely to conceive. By tracking ovulation, couples can pinpoint these fertile days and plan accordingly.
- **Seeking Medical Assistance:** If ovulation tracking and timed intercourse do not result in pregnancy after several months, it may be necessary to seek medical assistance. A fertility specialist can provide further guidance and perform tests to identify any underlying issues that may be affecting fertility.

Overall, tracking ovulation is a valuable tool for couples who are trying to conceive. By utilizing methods such as basal body temperature charting, cervical mucus observation, ovulation predictor kits, and smartphone apps, couples can enhance their understanding of their fertility and increase their chances of achieving pregnancy. Remember, every woman's journey to conception is unique, and it's important to consult with a healthcare professional for personalized advice and guidance.

Timing Intercourse

Timing intercourse plays a crucial role in maximizing the chances of conception. It is essential to understand the concept of the fertile window, which includes the days leading up to ovulation and the day of ovulation itself.

The fertile window refers to the period when a woman is most likely to conceive. Sperm can survive in the female reproductive system for up to five days, while the egg is viable for about 24 hours after ovulation. Therefore, having intercourse in the days leading up to ovulation increases the chances of sperm being present when the egg is released.

Tracking ovulation can help determine the timing of intercourse during the fertile window. Methods such as basal body temperature charting, cervical mucus observation, and ovulation predictor kits can provide valuable insights into the timing of ovulation. By identifying the most fertile days within the menstrual cycle, couples can plan intercourse accordingly and optimize their chances of conception.

Fertility Windows

Understanding the concept of fertility windows is crucial for maximizing the chances of conception. Fertility windows refer to the specific period within a woman's menstrual cycle when she is most likely to get pregnant. By tracking ovulation, women can identify these fertile days and plan intercourse accordingly.

During a typical menstrual cycle, ovulation usually occurs around the 14th day, counting from the first day of the menstrual period. However, this can vary from woman to woman and even from cycle to cycle. It is important to note that sperm can survive in the female reproductive system for up to five days, while the egg is viable for about 24 hours after ovulation. This means that the fertile window extends beyond the day of ovulation itself.

Tracking ovulation can help pinpoint the most fertile days within the menstrual cycle. There are several methods available for tracking ovulation, such as basal body temperature charting, cervical mucus observation, ovulation predictor kits, and smartphone apps. Each method has its own advantages and may be more suitable for different individuals.

By understanding the concept of fertility windows and utilizing effective ovulation tracking methods, women can increase their chances of conception and optimize their family planning. It is important to remember that fertility windows can vary from woman to woman and may be influenced by factors such as age, hormonal imbalances, and underlying medical conditions. Seeking medical assistance if needed and discussing fertility concerns with a healthcare professional can provide further guidance and support.

When to Seek Medical Assistance

When it comes to fertility concerns, seeking medical assistance can be crucial for couples trying to conceive. While ovulation tracking is a valuable tool in determining the most fertile days within a woman's menstrual cycle, it is not always a guarantee of pregnancy. If ovulation tracking alone does not result in pregnancy after several months of trying, it may be time to consider seeking medical assistance.

There are several situations in which it is recommended to seek medical assistance for fertility concerns. These include:

- **Advanced maternal age:** Women over the age of 35 may experience a decline in fertility, and it is generally recommended to seek medical advice after six months of trying to conceive.
- **Irregular menstrual cycles:** If a woman has irregular menstrual cycles, it may indicate an underlying hormonal imbalance or other medical condition that could affect ovulation. Seeking medical assistance can help identify and address these issues.

- **Known fertility issues:** If either partner has a known fertility issue, such as a history of reproductive disorders or previous difficulty conceiving, it is advisable to seek medical guidance sooner rather than later.
- **Unexplained infertility:** If ovulation tracking and timed intercourse have been consistently practiced for at least a year without success, it may be time to consult a fertility specialist to investigate potential causes of unexplained infertility.

It is important to remember that seeking medical assistance does not necessarily mean that fertility treatments or interventions will be immediately recommended. Often, medical professionals will conduct a thorough evaluation of both partners' reproductive health and provide guidance on optimizing fertility naturally. They may also suggest additional tests or treatments if necessary.

Ultimately, the decision to seek medical assistance for fertility concerns is a personal one. It is essential to communicate openly with your partner and healthcare provider to determine the best course of action for your unique situation. Remember, there is no shame in seeking help when it comes to building a family, and medical advancements have made it possible for many couples to overcome fertility challenges and fulfill their dreams of parenthood.

Conclusion

By understanding the basics of ovulation tracking, women can take control of their reproductive health, increase their chances of conception, and make informed decisions about family planning.

Ovulation tracking is a valuable tool for women who are trying to conceive. By monitoring their menstrual cycles and tracking ovulation, women can identify their most fertile days and time intercourse accordingly. This knowledge allows them to optimize their chances of conception and increase the likelihood of a successful pregnancy.

Furthermore, understanding ovulation can also help women manage their reproductive health. By tracking ovulation, women can identify any irregularities in their menstrual cycles or potential hormonal imbalances. This information can be shared with healthcare providers, enabling them to make accurate diagnoses and develop appropriate treatment plans if necessary.

In addition to aiding conception and reproductive health management, ovulation tracking also empowers women to make informed decisions about family planning. By knowing their fertile window and understanding their menstrual cycles, women can plan pregnancies more effectively. This knowledge can be particularly helpful for those who are trying to conceive or those who wish to avoid pregnancy.

Overall, ovulation tracking is a powerful tool that puts women in control of their reproductive health. By understanding the intricacies of their menstrual cycles and monitoring ovulation, women can increase their chances of conception, manage their reproductive health, and make informed decisions about family planning.

Frequently Asked Questions

- **Q: What is ovulation and why is it important?**

  A: Ovulation is the release of an egg from the ovary, which is a crucial step in the menstrual cycle for conception. It is important because it is the time when a woman is most fertile and has the highest chance of getting pregnant.

- **Q: How can I track my ovulation?**

  A: There are several methods to track ovulation, including basal body temperature charting, observing changes in cervical mucus, using ovulation predictor kits, and utilizing smartphone apps designed for ovulation tracking.

- **Q: What is basal body temperature charting?**

  A: Basal body temperature charting involves taking your temperature every morning before getting out of bed and recording it on a chart. It helps identify the slight rise in body temperature that occurs after ovulation, indicating that ovulation has already taken place.

- **Q: How can changes in cervical mucus help track ovulation?**

  A: Cervical mucus changes throughout the menstrual cycle, becoming clear, slippery, and stretchy around the time of ovulation. By observing these changes, you can determine when you are most fertile.

- **Q: How do ovulation predictor kits work?**

  A: Ovulation predictor kits detect the surge of luteinizing hormone (LH) in urine, which occurs one to two days before ovulation. They provide a positive result when the LH surge is detected, indicating that ovulation is likely to occur within the next 24 to 36 hours.

- **Q: Are smartphone apps reliable for tracking ovulation?**

  A: Smartphone apps can be reliable for tracking ovulation if they are designed with accurate algorithms and data input. However, it is important to choose a reputable app and use it in conjunction with other tracking methods for more accurate results.

- **Q: Is it true that every woman ovulates on day 14 of their cycle?**

A: No, the notion that every woman ovulates on day 14 is a misconception. The timing of ovulation can vary from woman to woman and even from cycle to cycle. It is important to track your own ovulation patterns to determine the most fertile days.

- **Q: Can irregular menstrual cycles affect ovulation tracking?**

A: Yes, irregular menstrual cycles can make it more challenging to track ovulation. It is important to adapt tracking methods to accommodate variations in cycle length and seek medical advice if irregularities persist.

- **Q: Do all women ovulate?**

A: No, not all women ovulate. Conditions such as anovulation can prevent ovulation from occurring regularly or at all. It is important to consult a healthcare professional if you have concerns about ovulation and fertility.

- **Q: What are the signs and symptoms of ovulation?**

A: Signs and symptoms of ovulation can include changes in cervical mucus consistency, ovulation pain (mittelschmerz), breast tenderness, increased libido, and changes in basal body temperature. These indicators can vary from woman to woman.

- **Q: Can stress affect ovulation?**

  A: Yes, stress can impact ovulation by disrupting the hormonal balance in the body. It is important to manage stress levels through relaxation techniques and self-care to optimize ovulation and fertility.

- **Q: How does age affect ovulation?**

  A: As women age, the frequency and quality of ovulation can decline. Fertility decreases as women approach their late 30s and 40s. It is important to be aware of these changes and seek medical advice if experiencing difficulties conceiving.

- **Q: When should I seek medical assistance for fertility concerns?**

  A: If ovulation tracking alone does not result in pregnancy after several months of trying, it may be necessary to seek medical assistance. A healthcare professional can provide guidance, perform tests, and recommend appropriate treatments to improve fertility.

Have Questions / Comments?

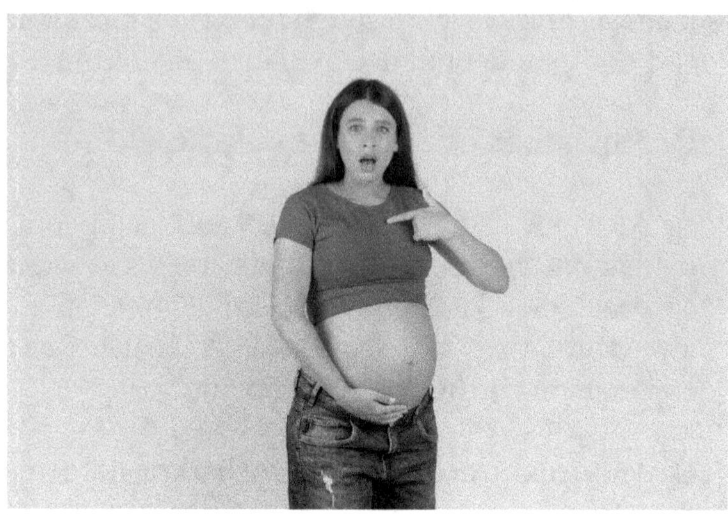

This book was designed to cover as much info as possible but I know I have probably missed something, or some new amazing discovery that has just come out.

If you notice something missing or have a question that I failed to answer, please get in touch and let me know. If I can, I will email you an answer and also update the book so others can also benefit from it.

Thanks For Being Awesome :)

Submit Your Questions / Comments At:

Get In Touch at Babydreamers.net

Get How To Be A Super Mom - 100% FREE

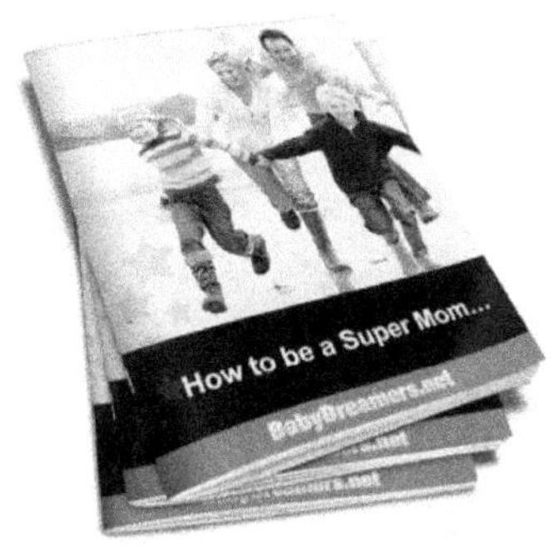

For being one of our amazing readers, we would love to offer you another book we have created, 100% free.

Being a mom is probably the most important job in the world – we've all heard that, and it's true. You're bringing up the next generation of wonderful, intelligent, loving, creative, responsible people.

We all want to be Super Mom and to be everything and do everything, but it this possible?

Being a Super Mom is possible, but you have to learn how to empower yourself to be the kind of Super Mom that you feel you need to be, keeping in mind that the title Super Mom doesn't mean the same thing to everyone.

Get How to be a Super Mom For Free at

BabyDreamers.net